IF YOU *Believe* IN YOURSELF

Anything IS POSSIBLE

Table of Contents

This book is written for those seeking for ways to shed some pounds and get into shape within the shortest possible time. Most times we find it difficult to squeeze out some time to hit the gym owing to our tight schedules. In this piece of well-crafted article, I will be giving out tips that will enable mothers and working class ladies to exercise at home at their convenience.

I have taken out time to research and analyze a couple of exercises which I have drafted into a menu with daily sets of exercises. In addition to this, I have prepared a few nutritional procedures. If you follow this menu judiciously, you will certainly experience great reformation and will certainly lose lots of pounds with a limited time frame.

And a few word about proper nutrition.

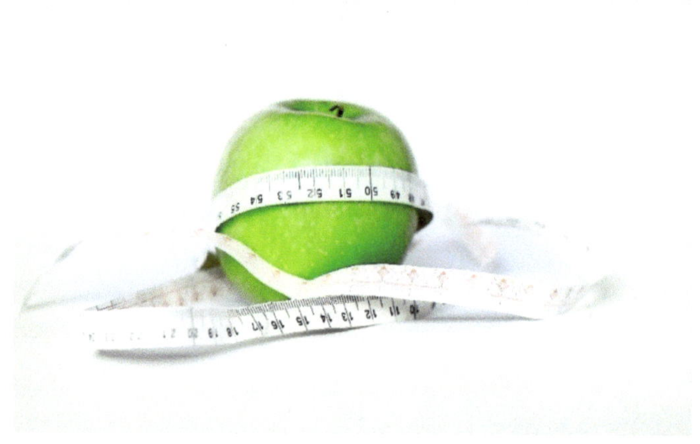

You Need To Know About Maintaining Proper Nutrition in Your Diet

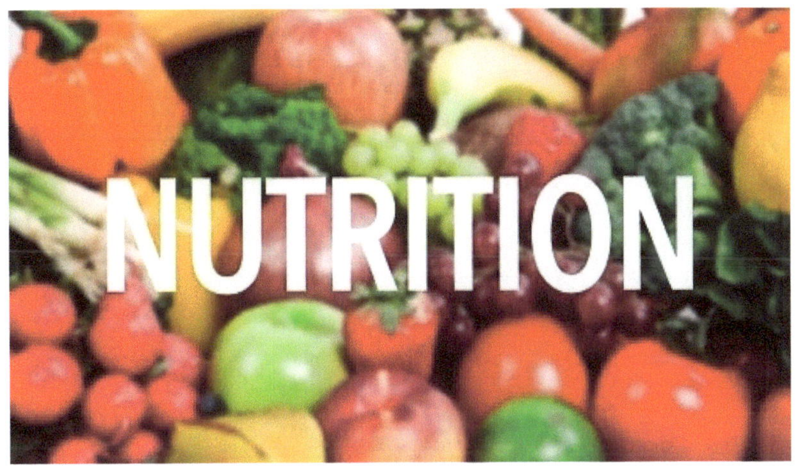

Are you aiming at leading a healthy life? If you are, then you need to subscribe to a healthy lifestyle. It is very simple and beneficial in so many ways. Ten percent depends on your genetics, ten percent on the exercises you do, and eighty percent on your diet. Some of the main benefits of engaging in a healthy lifestyle include:

- Controlling your weight- In order to lose weight, you need to regulate your calorie intake. This includes making sure that you do not consume more calories than you are going to burn within a day. This helps you prevent weight-related diseases and conditions such as obesity, clogged arteries, cardiovascular diseases, thyroid dysfunction, and even type-2 diabetes.

- Improving brain performance- Subscribing to proper nutrition boosts the flow of blood that goes to the brain. This improves brain functionalities and helps prevent the development of Alzheimer's disease.

- Boost energy levels in the body- This will provide you with enough energy to go through your daily routine. Stick to eating unprocessed carbohydrates like vegetables, fruits, and even whole grains.

- Strengthening your teeth and bones- This is through a steady intake of calcium in your diet form fortified foods a low-fat dairy product.

- Boosts the health of your heart- This is by reducing your intake of sodium, cholesterol, and fats.

Healthy Eating Habits You Need To Practice

To attain this optimum status of proper nutrition, you need to regulate and monitor your consumption of nutrients. This means that on a daily basis:

1. Twenty to thirty-five percent of your intake should consist of fats
2. Ten to thirty-five percent should consist of protein
3. Forty-five to sixty-five percent should consist of carbohydrates

Other than this, you need to practice healthy eating habits. They include:

- Increasing the intake of energy giving foods and proteins when engaging in sport and other high-energy activities
- Instead of limiting yourself to three bulky meals a day, you need to eat five-six small meals. These will help keep you satiated and prevent you from consuming calorie-filled foods. Thus, make sure

that you have breakfast, lunch, supper, one snack before bed, and two snacks during the day.

- Drink a lot of water. Instead of limiting yourself to the average eight to ten glasses a day, try drinking water every time you feel thirsty. Drink a glass of water before you eat, this will help you regulate your food portions and prevent you from increasing your calorie intake

- If you are about to engage in an active sport, eat after the activity is complete. Eating before the game will definitely affect your metabolism. Thus, try eating a heavy meal in the morning and a snack right before the sport. Eating afterward will help you replenish your energy level.

Following the above precautions and guidelines will definitely help you kick-start a healthy lifestyle. You will see the results after a short period if you practice patience and persistence.

About The Program

During the course of this program, desist from consuming sweets, flour, fried and fatty foods. If you are in the habit of eating 5 meals a day, and you cannot find the meal routine on the given menu list, kindly replace any not found with another one from the next or previous day's menu. Avoid eating fruits once it is 14:00 and if you must eat, make sure it isn't above 250 grams.

Drink adequate amount of water: Drink lots of water during the day and also between exercises. Drink at least 30 ml of water per kg of your weight. This will aid in quenching your taste, and in energizing you during exercises.

Outfits: As a lady, you will need to put on clothes that will make you feel comfortable. Leggings are ideal wears to be worn over a pair of t-shirts or sports bras. Low impact exercising shoes such as sneakers should be worn to protect your feet.

Exercises: It's pretty natural to experience difficulties during the first three days of an exercise but with persistence and patience, you will overcome such challenges. To achieve adequate results, each individual will be given a specific time frame to finish an assignment. It doesn't matter if you spend some 30minutes, 40 minutes or an hour trying to complete a given task; the most important thing is completing the task. While exercising, monitor your heart rate with varying degrees of intensity training. The table below can serve as a guide.

Caution: stop if you feel faint, dizzy or exhausted.

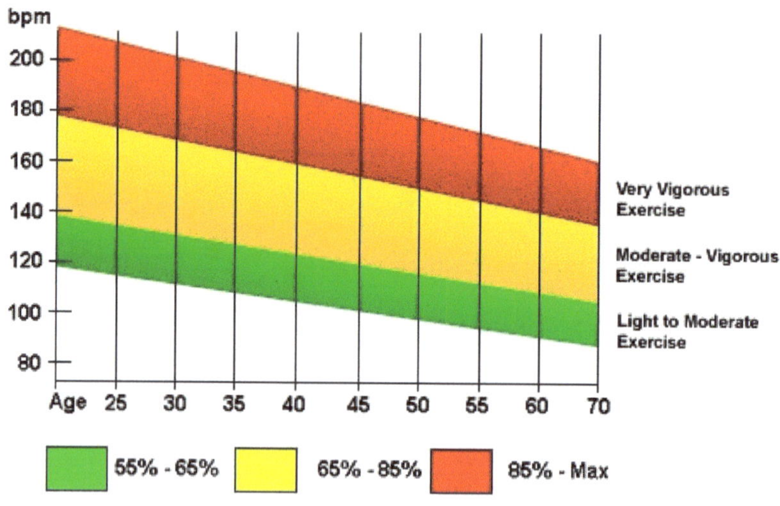

Things To Do Before And After Training

Before training: Before commencing with your workout, ensure you wash your face in order to wash off any cosmetics on your face. This is because, during workout, the sweat and sebaceous glands become agitated thereby making it prone to infections. Hence, for a face with a makeup, the contaminated sweats can easily enter the eyes which could be harmful to it.

After training: Hit the bathroom and have a warm shower. If after having your bath, your skin feels dry, apply your body cream or lotion to moisturize your skin. Endeavor to wash our face with a cleansing tonic, as this will help the skin to get toned up easily. If you do not adhere to these simple procedures, there is the possibility of pimples appearing on your face.

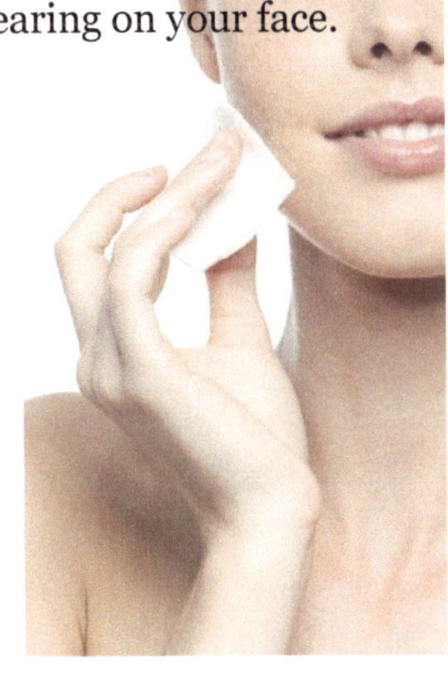

Menu day 1

(menu at 1500-1600 kcal)

For breakfast: brown rice (about 200 grams) + sandwich with cucumber caviar and whole-grain bread

For lunch: One baked apple + 20 pieces of almonds

For dinner: take about 200 grams of Pasta of any shape + a 100g of tuna juice

For afternoon snack you can take Curd with berries and honey.

Recipe: 200 g cottage cheese (0.1% fat) + a handful of any berries, and 1 tbsp. of honey

For supper: Any white baked fish with cucumber.

Exercises for Today
Warm-up

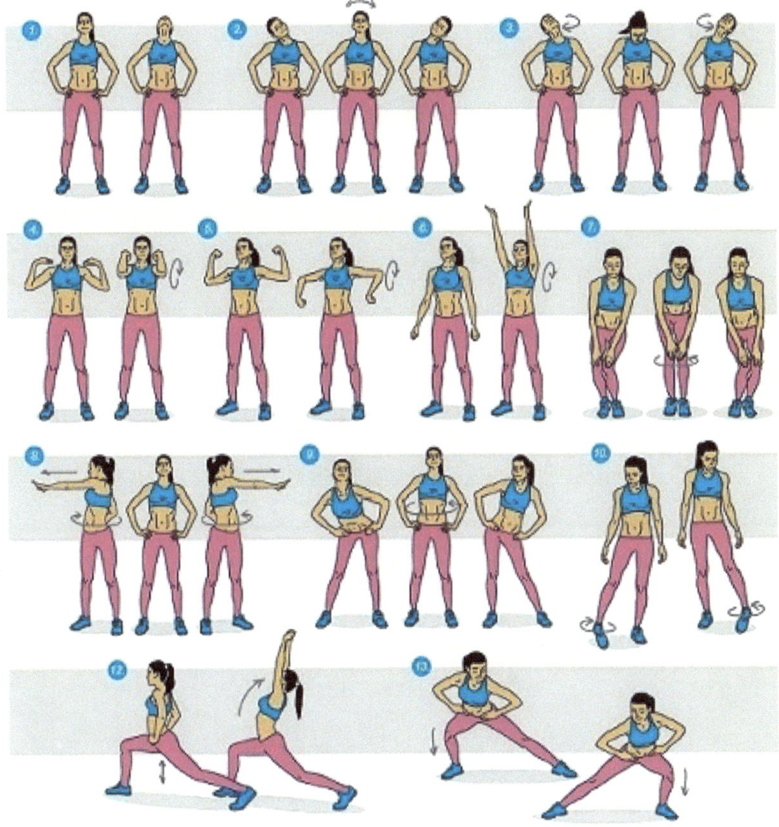

First block: 3 circles, rest between circles 30 sec, between blocks – 1 min

1 Jumping 30 sec

2 Push-ups 10 rep (if it's hard than push-ups from the knees)

3 Lunges with a side leg lift 15 rep (on each leg)

4 Running on the spot with the high raising of knees 30 sec

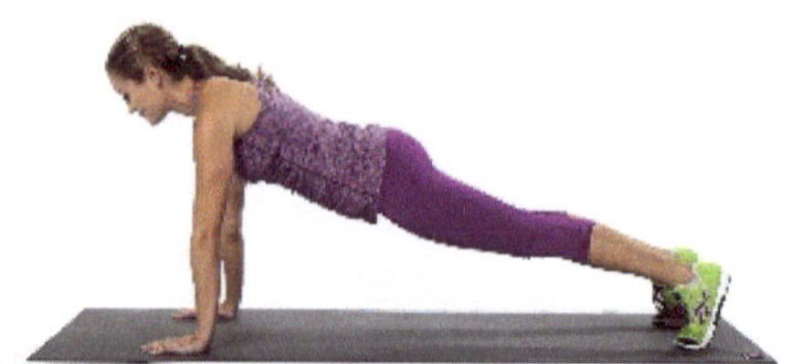

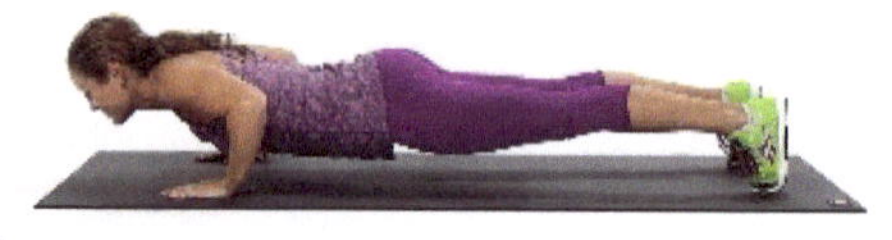

2

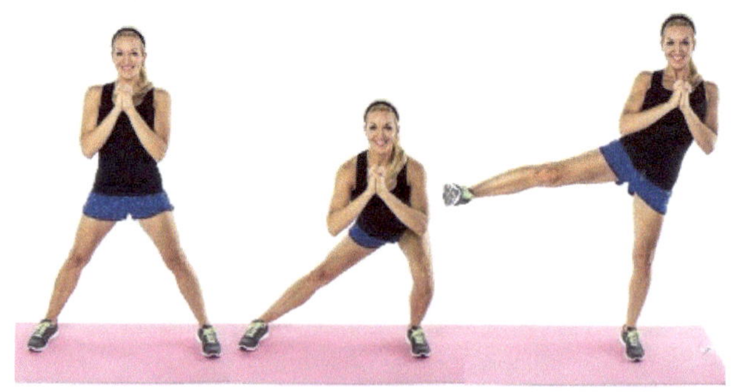

3

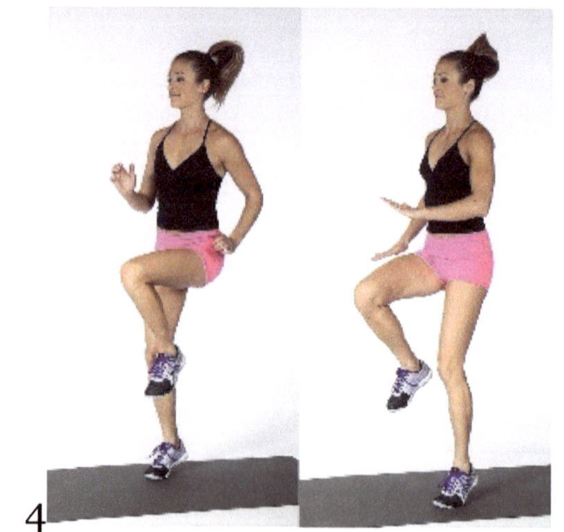

4

Copyright © 2018 by Daniela Shar

Second block: ***3 circles, rest between circles 30 sec***

5 Bicycle crunches 25 rep

6 Reverse crunches 20 rep

7 Floor hyperextension 25 rep

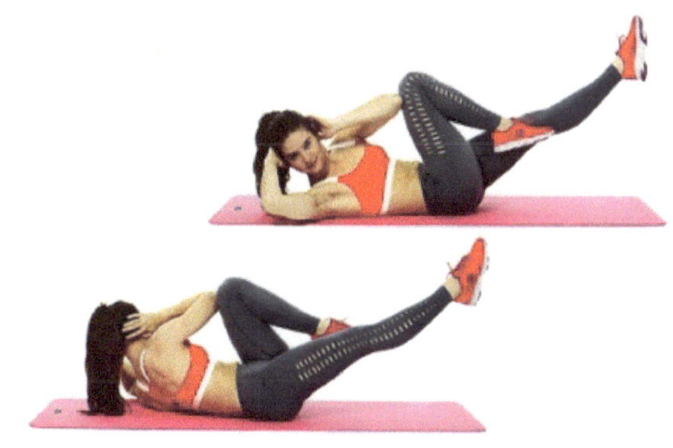

5

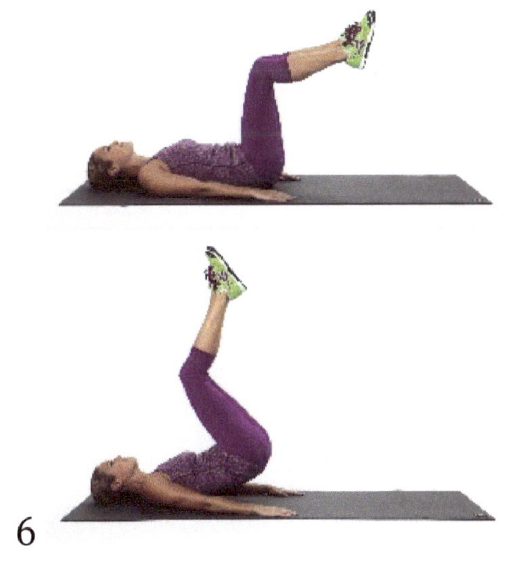

6

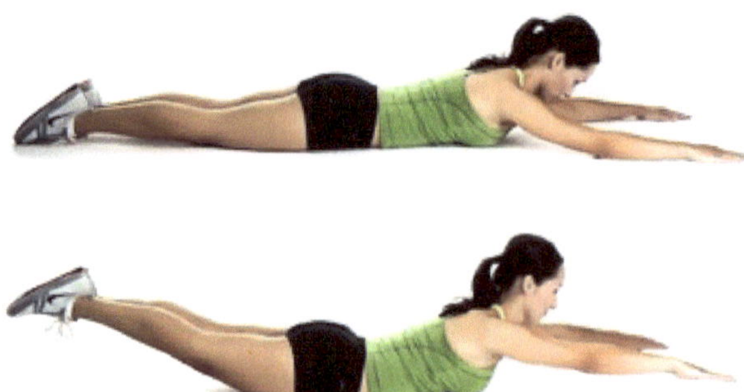

7

Menu day 2
(menu at 1500 -1600 kcal)

Breakfast: 200 grams of oatmeal, and 1 banana.

Snack: carrot salad.

Lunch: buckwheat or rice porridge, steam cutlet with vegetables.

Snack: 100 grams of berries or fruit salad (small portion, about half a glass).

Dinner: assorted vegetables, 200 grams of chicken breast.

Exercises for Today
Warm-up

First block: 3 circles, rest between circles 30 sec, between blocks – 1 min

1 Burpee 10 rep

2 Squats 20 rep

3 Jump lunges 10 rep

4 Plank-jacks 20 rep

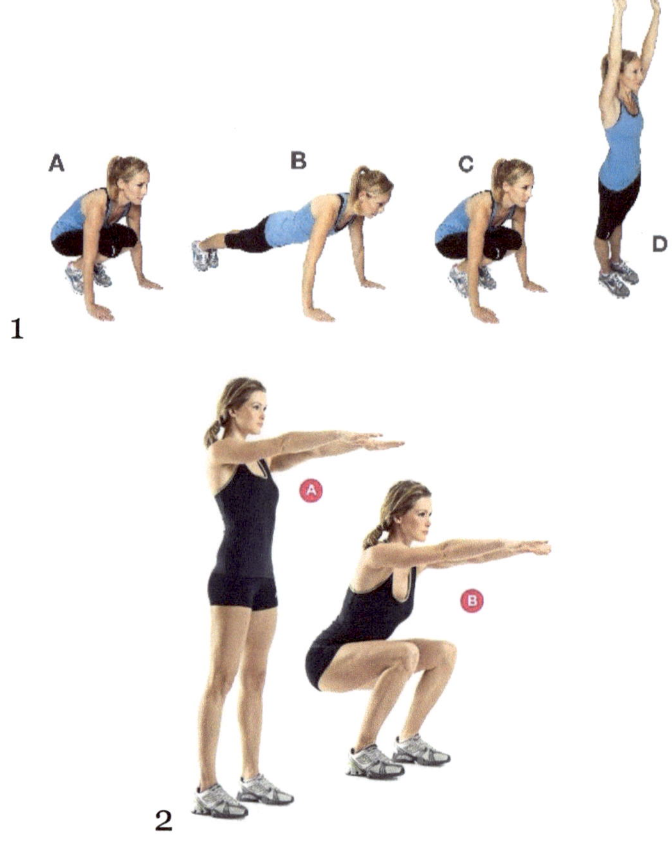
A
B
C
D
1
A
B
2

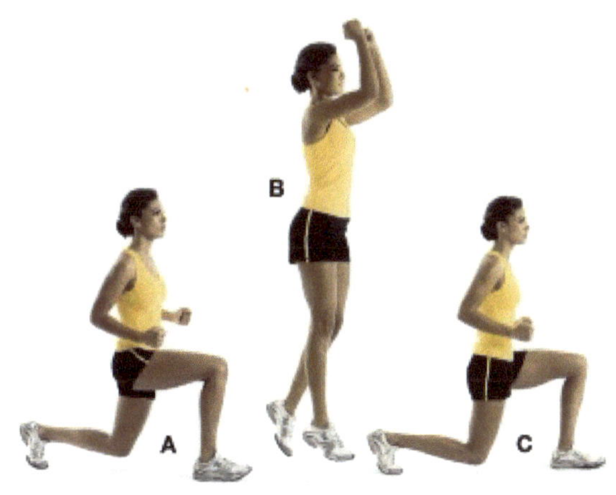

3

4

Second block: **3 circles, rest between circles 30 sec**

5 Crunches 20 rep

6 Russian twist crunches 30 rep

7 Plank hip dips 30 rep

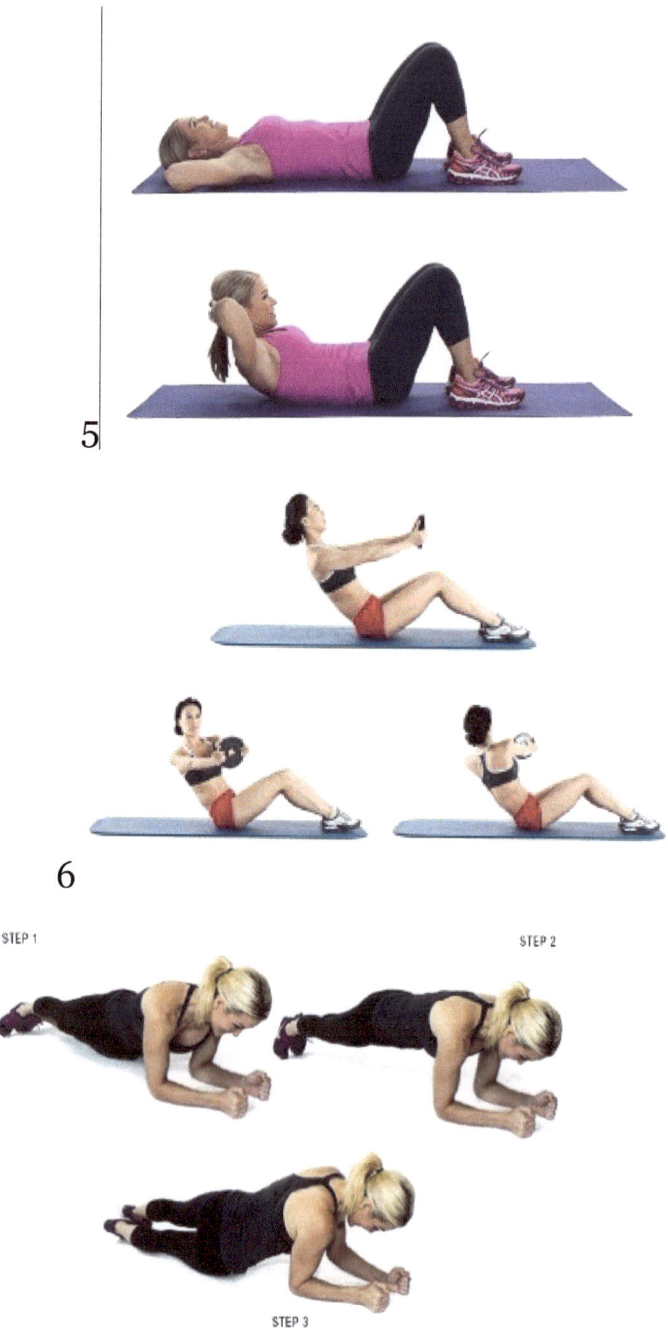

5
6
STEP 1
STEP 2
STEP 3
7

Menu day 3

(menu at 1550 -1650 kcal)

For breakfast: 50 grams of boiled bulgur (weight is considered in dry form) + add 2 teaspoons of dried fruits + 1 teaspoon of walnuts; 1 baked apple with 1 teaspoon of honey.

For lunch: A few thin slices of the breast of chicken wrapped in a thin sheet of pita bread 15x15 + greens, cucumber, 1 hard pear.

For dinner: soup with beets and cabbage (without meat broth) weighing about 200 g, 1 tablespoon of low-fat sour cream, 1 piece of rye bread with bran; 100 g of boiled fish with green peas 50 g.

For afternoon snack: low-fat cottage cheese (200 g) + 1 cup of kefir.

Exercises for Today
Warm-up

First block: 3 circles, rest between circles 30 sec, between blocks 1 min

1 Jumping jacks 30 rep

2 180-degree jump squats 20 rep

3 Push-ups 20 rep (if it's hard than push-ups from the knees)

4 Side plank leg lift 20 rep (20 rep on each leg)

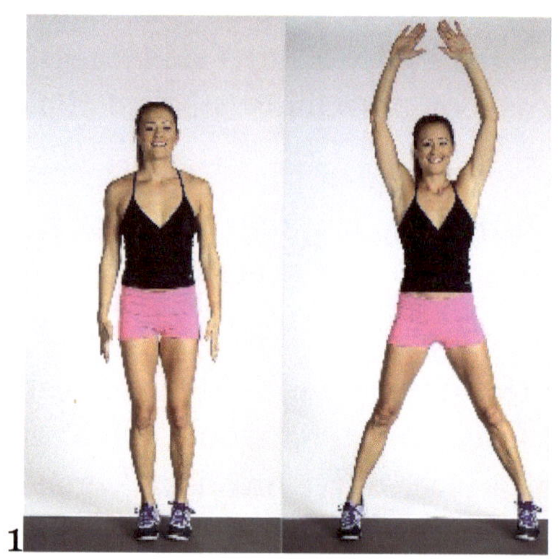

1

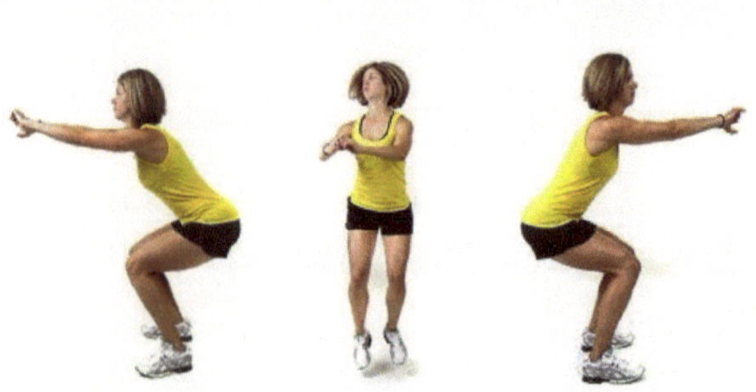

2

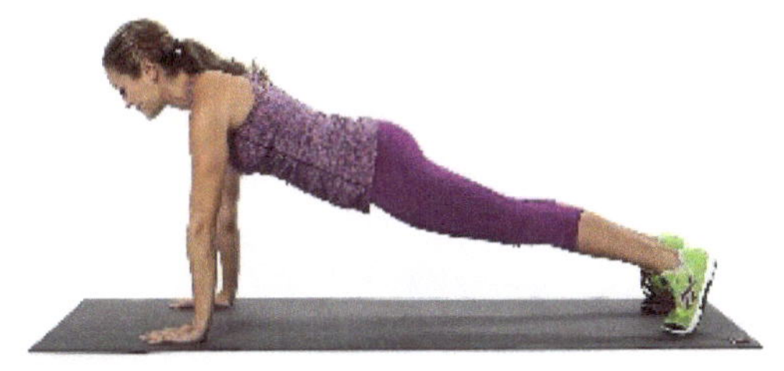

3   4

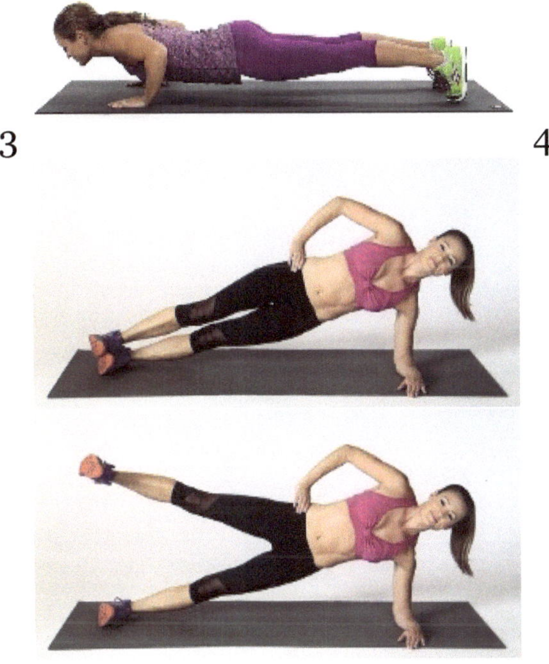

***Second block**: 3 circles, rest between circles 30 sec*

5 The V-sit crunches 25 rep

6 Scissor crunches 30 rep

7 Side plank with hip dips 30 rep (15 rep on each leg)

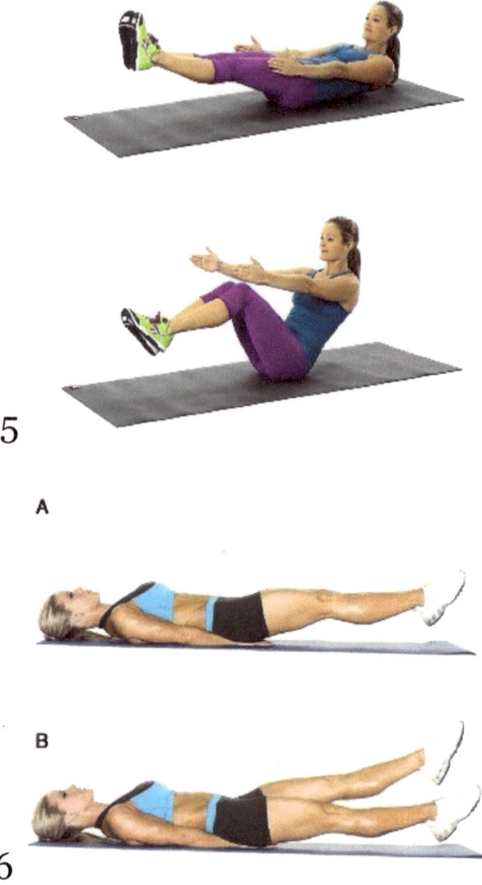

5

A

B

6

A

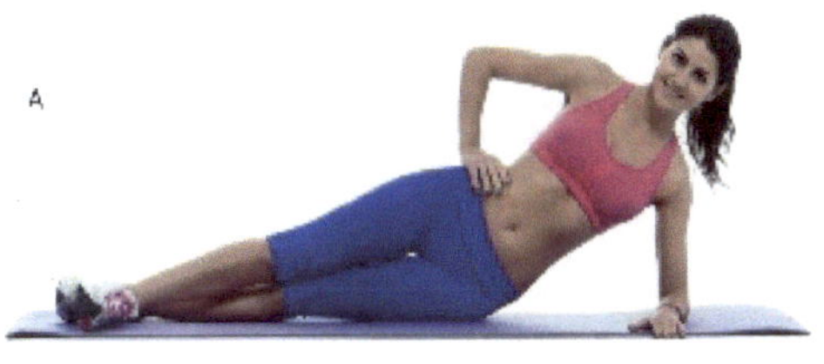

B

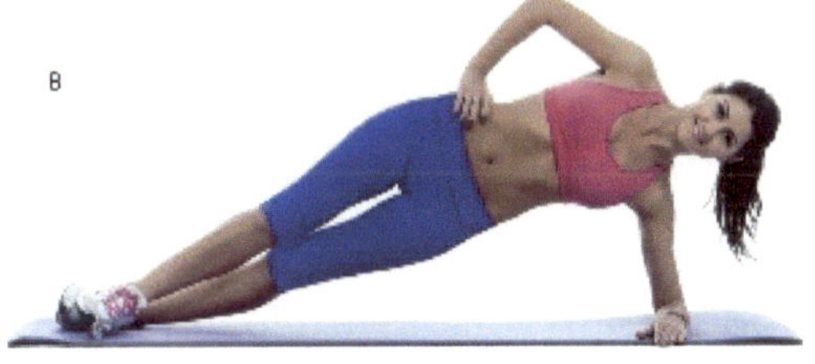

7

Menu day 4

(menu at 1500 -1600 kcal)

For breakfast: 1 small baked potato; 100 ml of milk 1,5% and 150 g of frozen berries whip mixed together; 2 toasted rye bread; 1 piece of cheese.

For lunch: whole-grain bread with low-fat cheese

For dinner: eat 180 grams of chicken meat without skin, stewed with chopped pepper, zucchini, carrots, onions and brown rice (2 tablespoons). Add 1 teaspoon of vegetable oil at the end of cooking and 1 cup of tomato juice.

For afternoon snack: 100 grams of cottage cheese + 1 tomato.

For supper you can make salad: boiled cabbage broccoli + cauliflower, lettuce leaves, 1/2 sweet pepper, olives, 1 boiled egg, 1 teaspoon of vegetable oil, lemon juice, spices, greens + 150 g of fish (baked or canned).

Drink a cup of kefir with 1% fat after 1 – 1.5 hours

Exercises for Today
Warm-up

First block: 3 circles, rest between circles 30 sec, between blocks – 1 min

1 Jump burpee 15 rep

2 Donkey kicks 40 rep (20 on each leg)

3 Plank-into-squats 20 rep

4 Boxing 40 min

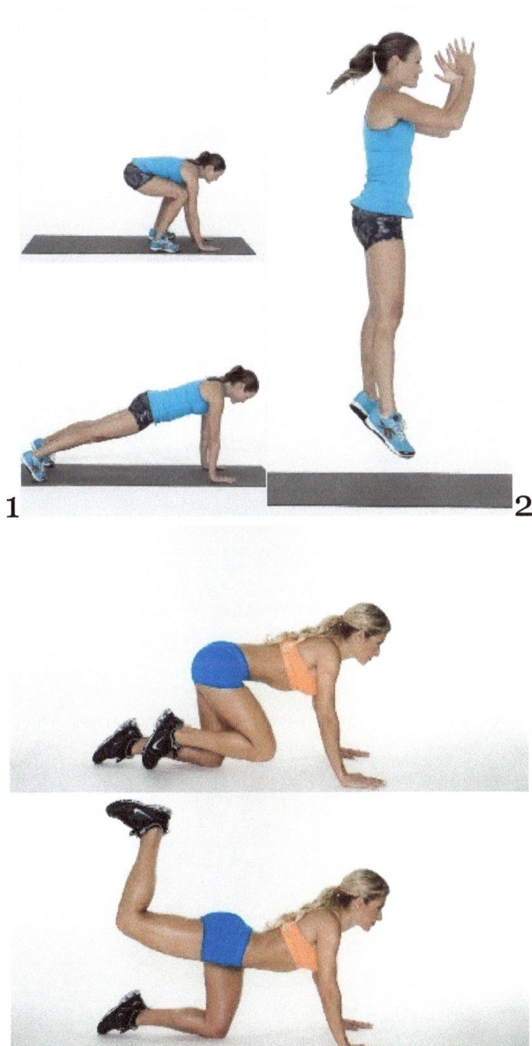

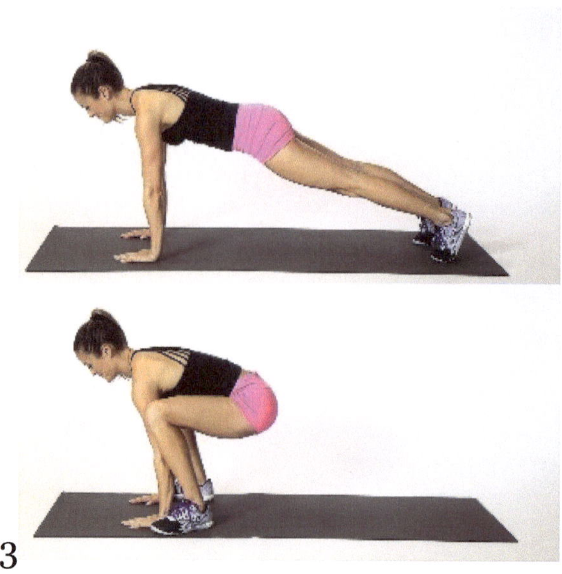

3

Second block: **_3 circles, rest between circles 30 sec_**

5 Full sit-up crunches 25 rep

6 Bicycle crunches 30 rep

7 Hyperextension on floor 25 rep

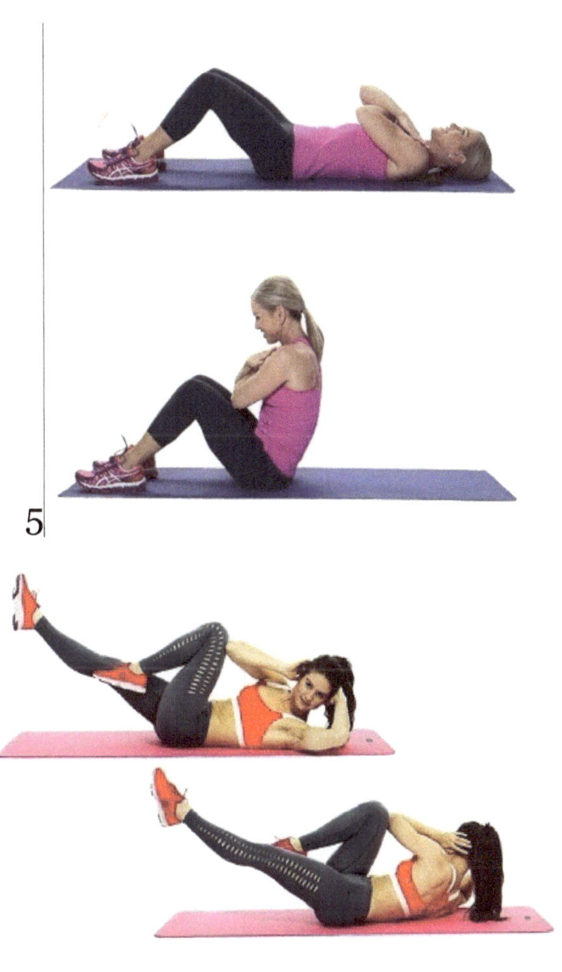

5

6

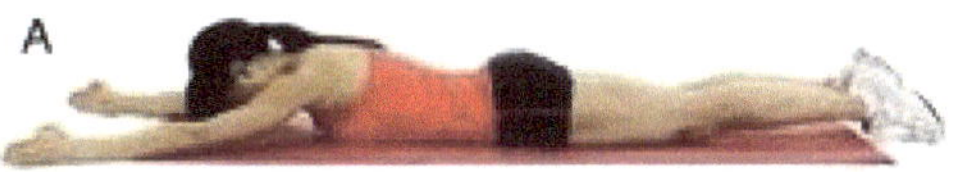

A

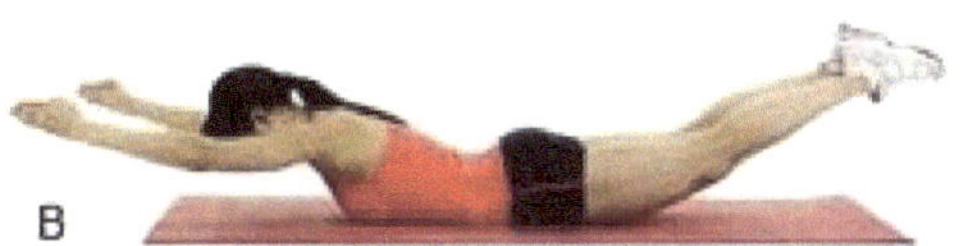

B

7

Menu day 5

(menu at 1400 -1500 kcal)

For breakfast: take about 200 grams of porridge brown rice, and some apple.

For snack: drink about 150 ml of low-fat natural yogurt or a glass of yogurt, and bread.

For lunch: mix and eat 100 grams of buckwheat, with 100 grams of boiled beef, and 200 grams of lettuce (tomato, cucumber, lettuce leaves).

For afternoon snack: take smoothies (mix 100 grams of cottage cheese or 1 banana, with 100 ml of milk and half a glass of berries together).

For dinner: eat 100 grams of steamed fish, with boiled asparagus, and grain loaf.

Exercises for Today
Warm-up

First block: 3 circles, rest between circles 30 sec, between blocks – 1 min

1 Burpees 20 rep

2 Squats with side rise leg 30 rep

3 Up-down plank 15 rep

4 Speed skaters 30 rep

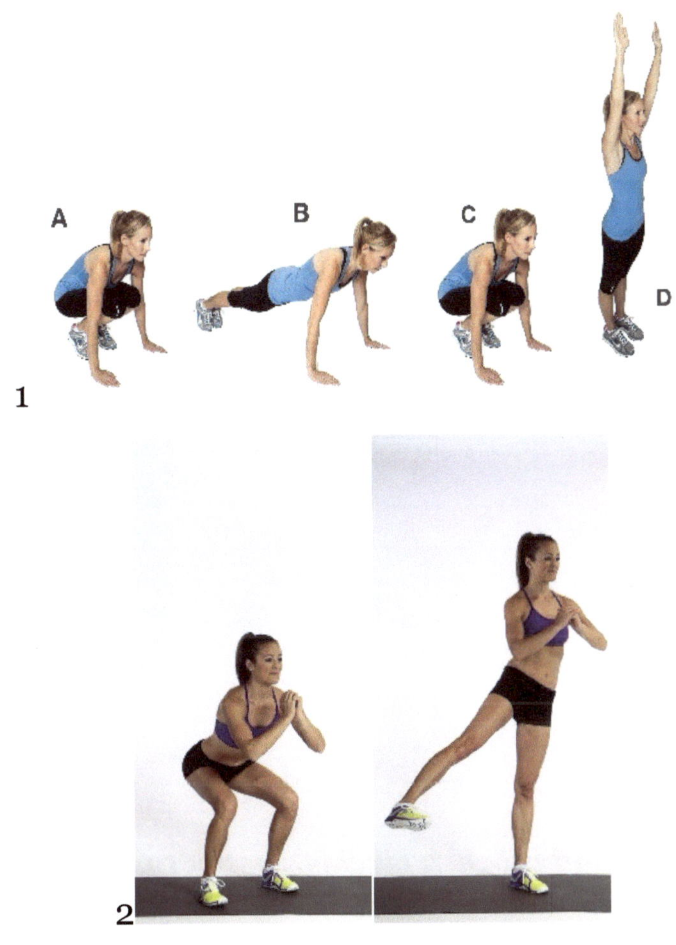

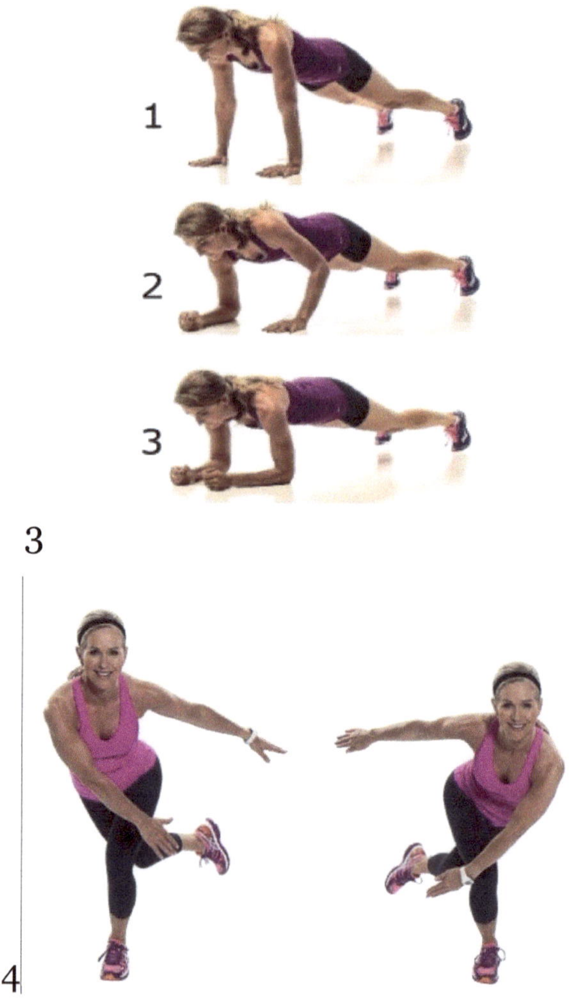

***Second block**: 3 circles, rest between circles 30 sec*

5 Mountain climber crunches 30 rep

6 Reverse crunches 25 rep

7 Seated knee crunches 30 rep

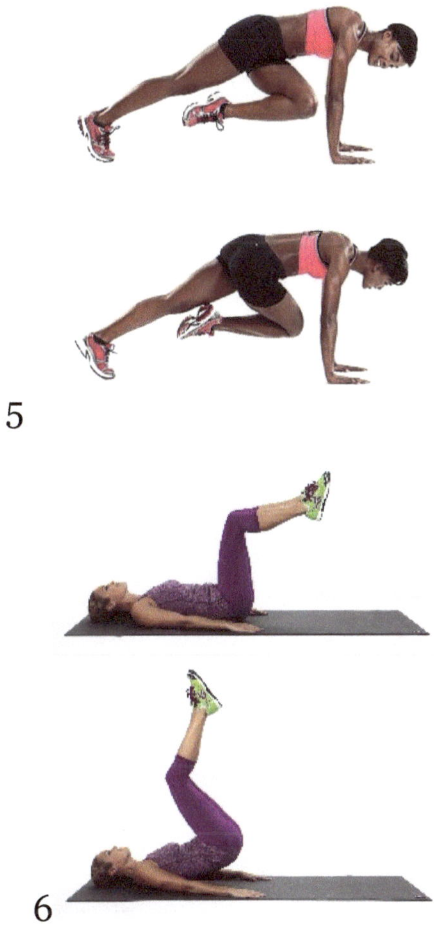

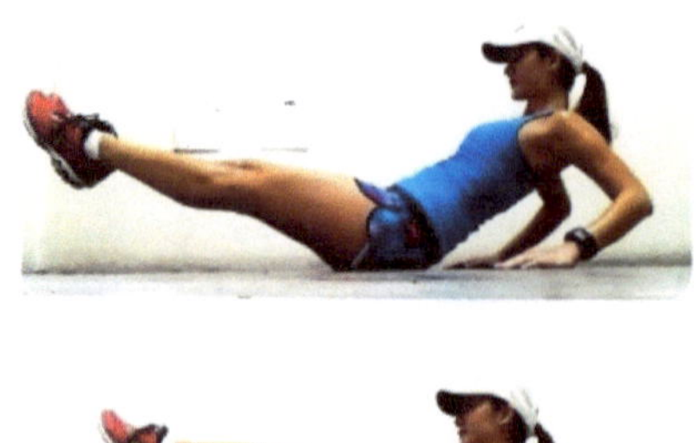

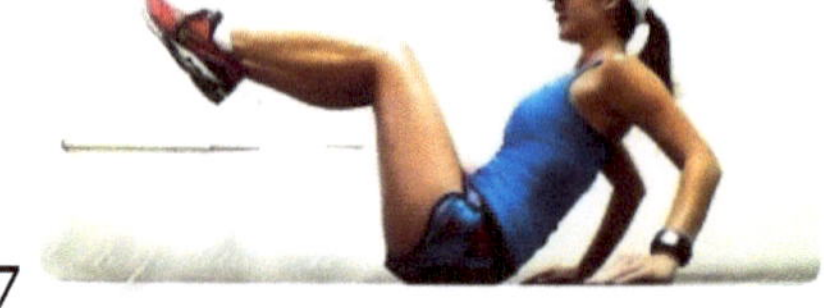

7

Menu day 6

(menu at 1400 -1500 kcal)

For breakfast: eat 200 g of oatmeal or muesli on skim milk, apple, and tea

For second breakfast: consume a reasonable quantity of carrot and apple salad

For lunch: eat vegetable soup, with a glass of juice

For snack: a toast of black bread with a slice of low-calorie cheese

For dinner: boiled chicken fillet - 100 grams, stewed vegetables with herbs - 300 g, 1 tbsp. kefir

Before going to bed: take a glass of herbal tea

Exercises for Today
Warm-up

First block: 3 circles, rest between circles 30 sec, between blocks – 1 min

1 Jumping jacks 35 rep

2 1 leg squat chair dip 30 rep (15 on each leg)

3 Plank jacks 20 rep

4 Running on the spot with the high raising of knees 40
sec

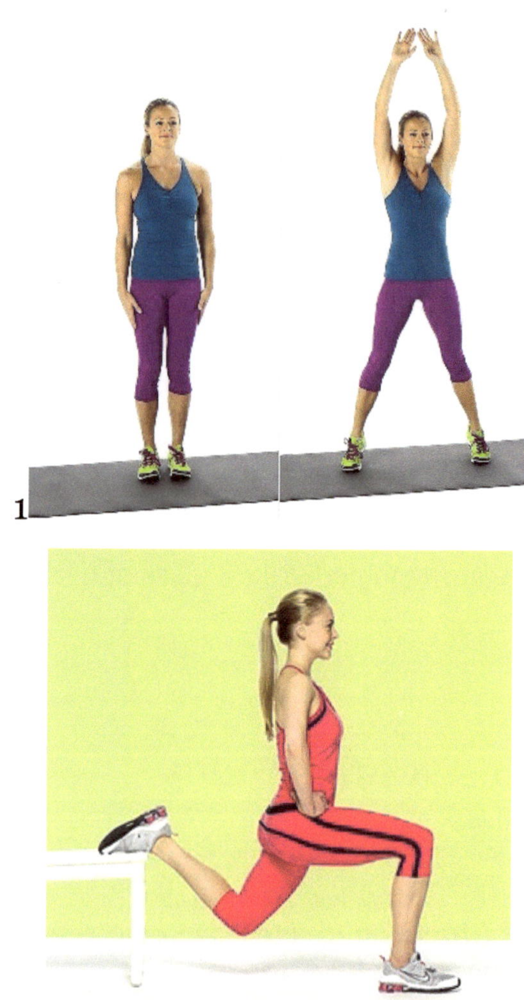

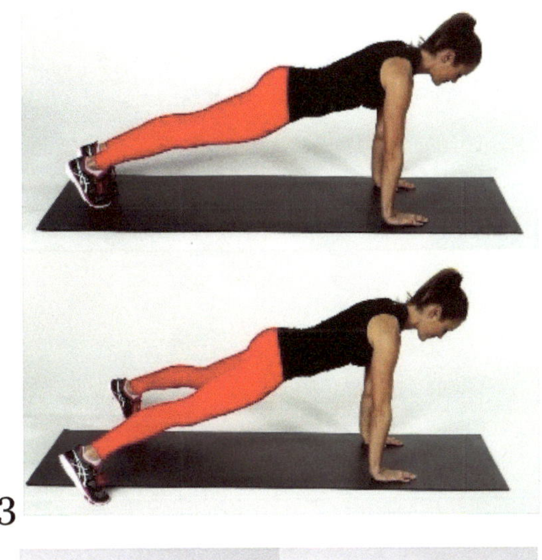

3

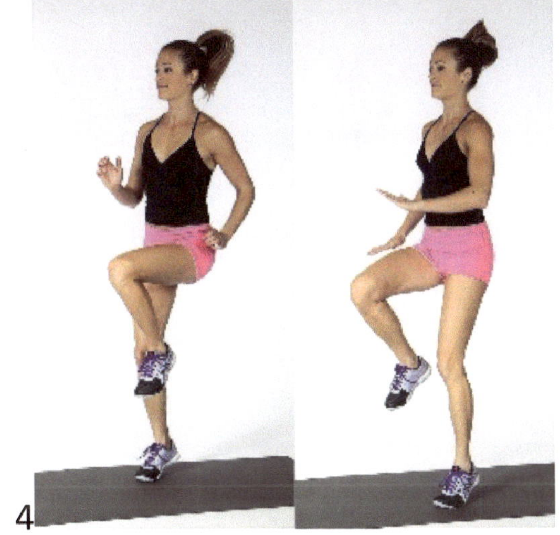

4

Second block*: *3 circles, rest between circles 30 sec

5 Crunches 30 rep

6 Scissors crunches 30 rep

7 Hip raises 40 rep

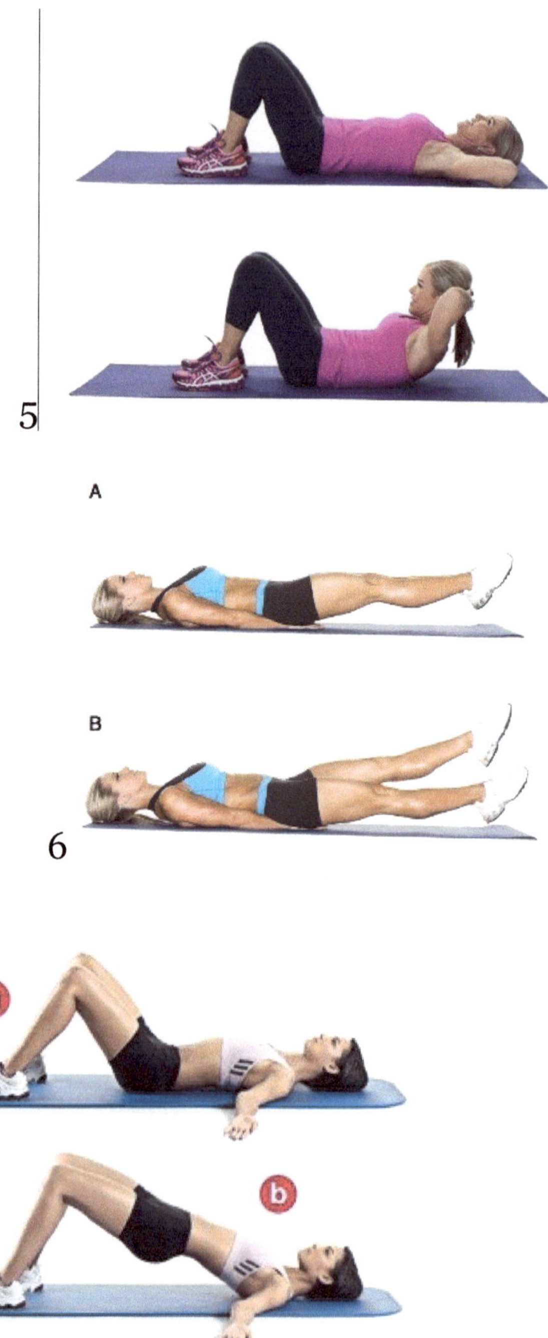

5
A
B
6
a
b
7

Menu day 7

(menu at 1400 -1500 kcal)

For breakfast: oatmeal

Recipe: Oat flakes (NOT fast cooking) plain yogurt without fillers or kefir glass jar with a lid of 0.5 or 0.4 liters. Add oatmeal, yogurt, some honey and your favorite fruit or berries. Close the jar with a lid and shake vigorously.

After breakfast, you can drink herbal or green tea

For snack: dilute 1% of 150 grams of curd with kefir and sweetened with stevia.

For dinner: brown rice or buckwheat + vegetables + 2 cutlets from chicken fillet baked or steamed

For lunch: omelet (2 eggs) + any vegetables (150 g)

For supper: fresh vegetable salad (250 g) + teaspoon of oil + baked or boiled lean meat (150 g)

Exercises for Today

Warm-up

First block: 3 circles, rest between circles 30 sec, between blocks – 1 min

1 Jump burpees 15 rep

2 180-degree jump squats 25 rep

3 Reverse lunge knee-up 40 rep (20 on each leg)

4 Boxing 40 sec

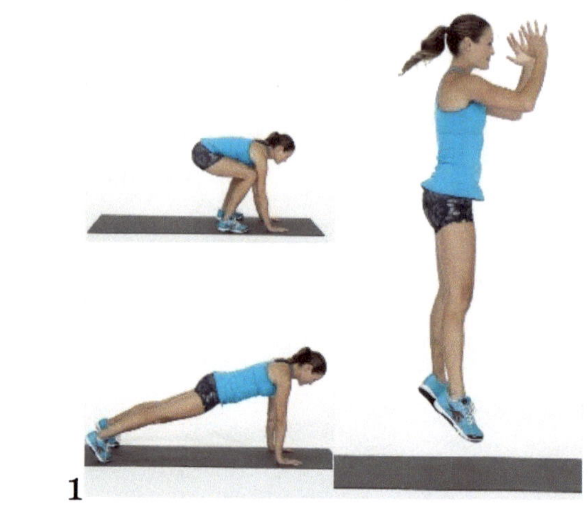

1

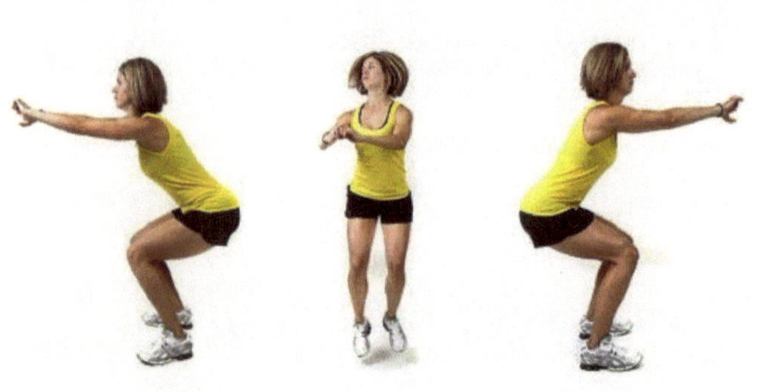

2

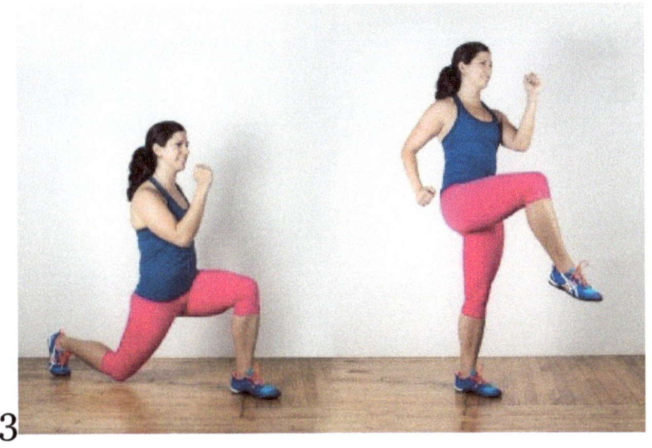

3

Second block: *3 circles, rest between circles 30 sec*

5 The V-sit crunches 30 rep

6 Russian twist crunches 30 rep

7 Standing crossover crunches 40 rep (20 on each leg)

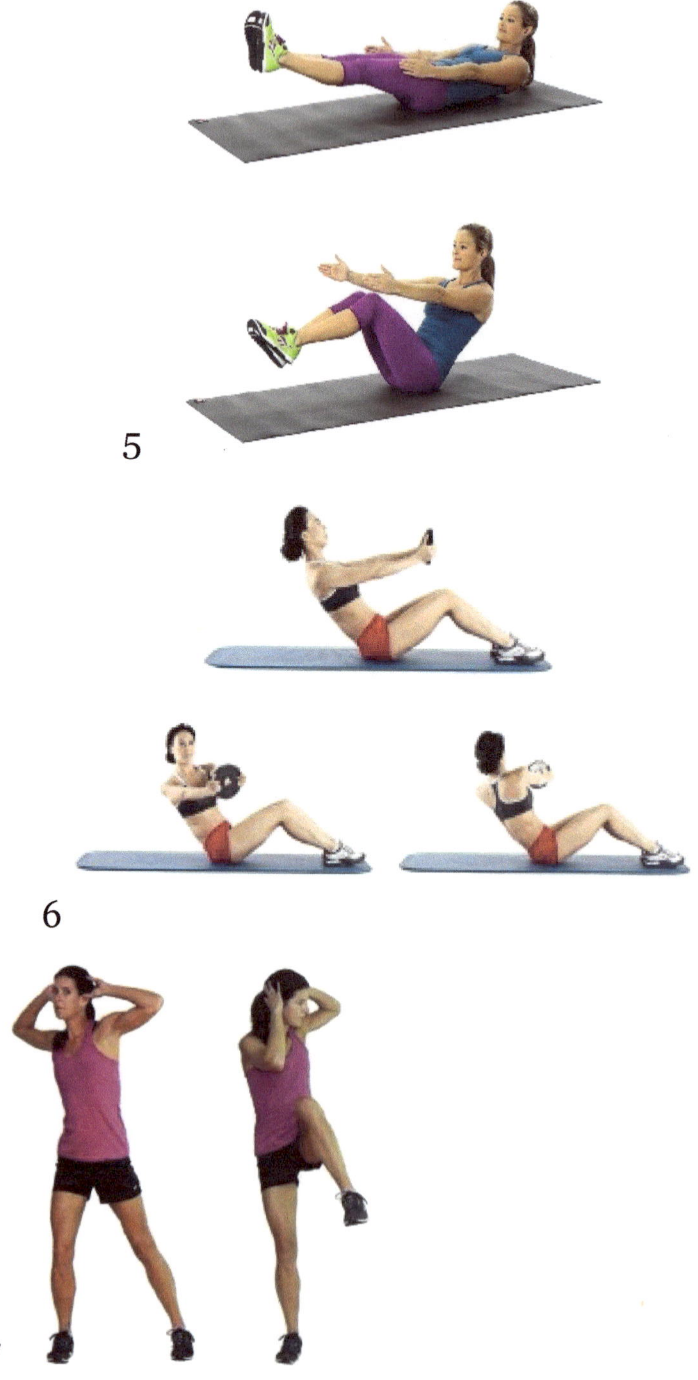

5

6

7

Menu day 8

(menu at 1400-1500 kcal)

For breakfast: *take* any cereal with 100 g dry milk + herbal or green tea.

For lunch: mix an orange, with a cup of cocoa and milk and eat it with a slice of bread and 1 teaspoon of honey.

For dinner: macaroni of solid varieties weighing 150 g / porridge pea / millet/buckwheat Beef/chicken goulash 100 g vegetable salad.

For snack: curd 150 gr + a handful of any berries, 1 tbsp. honey

For supper: Greek salad (tomatoes, cucumbers, peppers, olives, feta cheese) + baked low-fat meat or fish in the oven (150 g)

Exercises for Today
Warm-up

First block: 3 circles, rest between circles 30 sec, between blocks – 1 min

1 Burpee 20 rep

2 Squats with side rise leg 30 rep

3 Plank jacks 25 rep

4 Jumping 30 sec

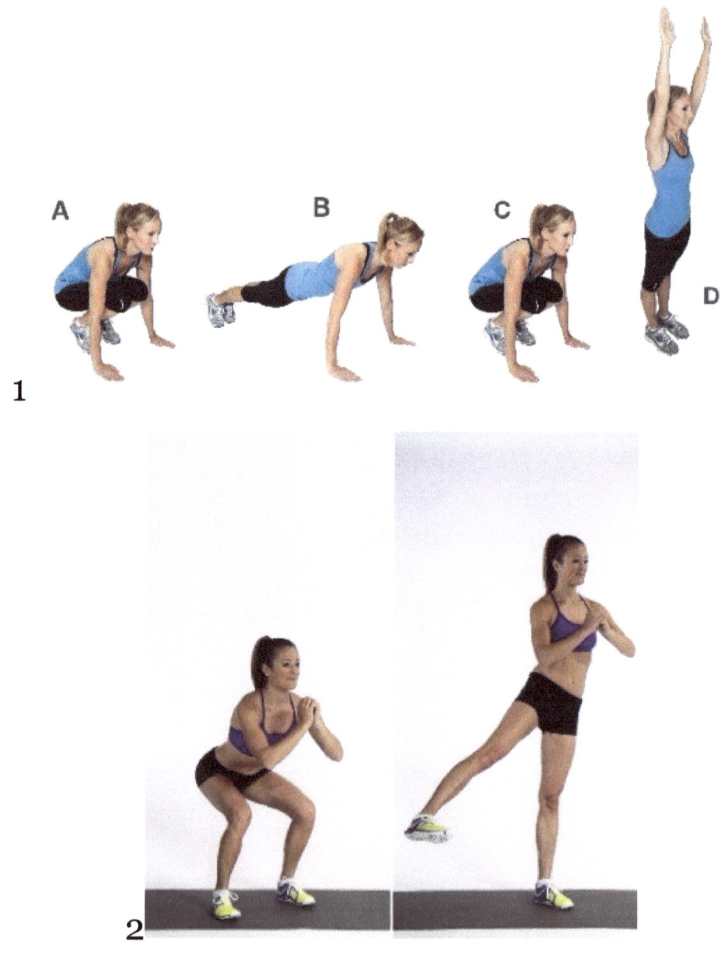

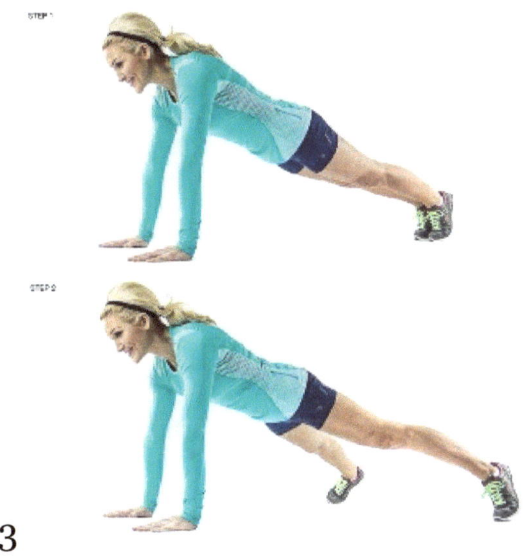

3

Second block: 3 circles, rest between circles 30 sec

5 Full sit-ups 30 rep

6 Mountain climber crunches 30 rep

7 Hyperextension on floor 30 rep

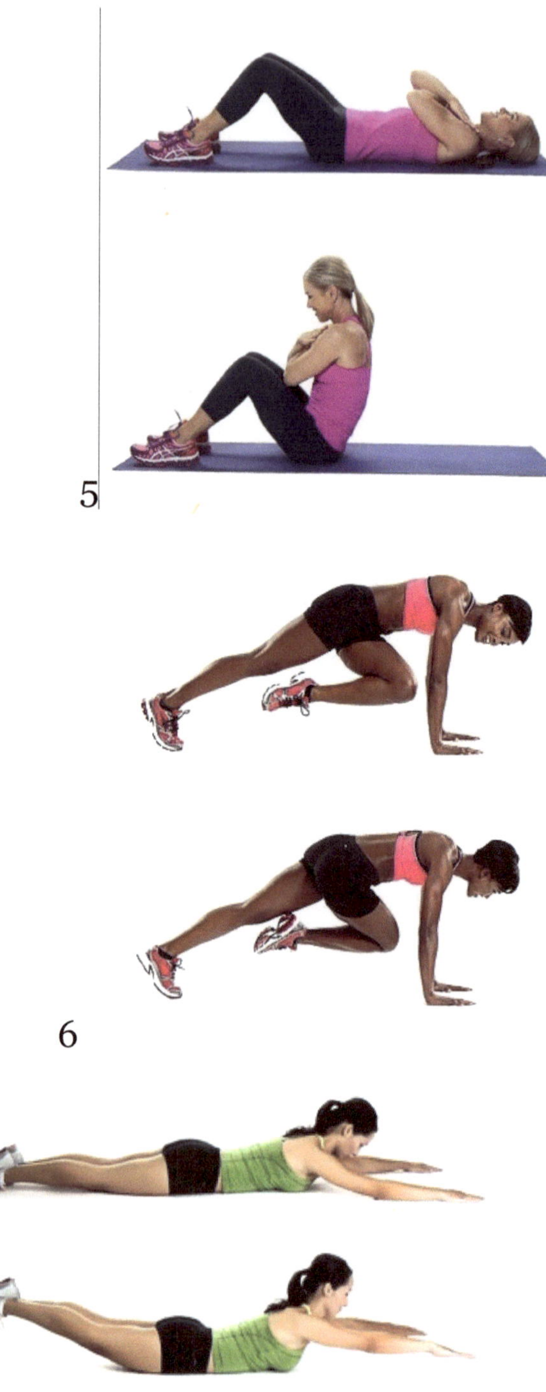

5

6

7

Menu day 9

(menu at 1400-1500 kcal)

For Breakfast: Make an Omelet from 2 eggs with greens using a half teaspoon of oil+ 50 grams of porridge (weight in dry form).

For drink, take herbal or green tea

For lunch: natural yogurt without additives and weighing 100 g + an apple or pear or 150 grams of berries or whole-grain bread with cheese

For dinner: vegetable soup (200 grams with potatoes, without meat broth) + bread with peanut butter

For snack: curd or kefir (150 grams) + cinnamon to taste

For supper: baked fish (white fish in the lemon marinade) with fresh vegetables without butter and dressing.

Exercises for Today
Warm-up

First block: 3 circles, rest between circles 30 sec, between blocks – 1 min

1 Jump burpees 20 rep

2 1 leg squat chair dip 30 rep (15 on each leg)

3 push-ups 20 rep (if it's hard than push-ups from the knees)

4 Boxing 40 sec

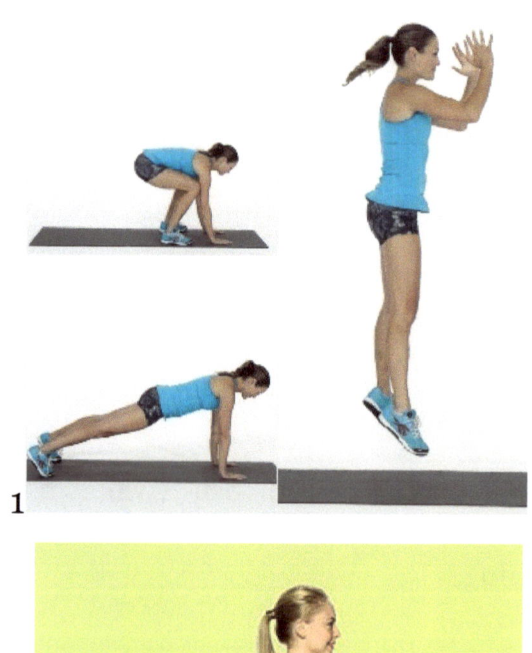

1

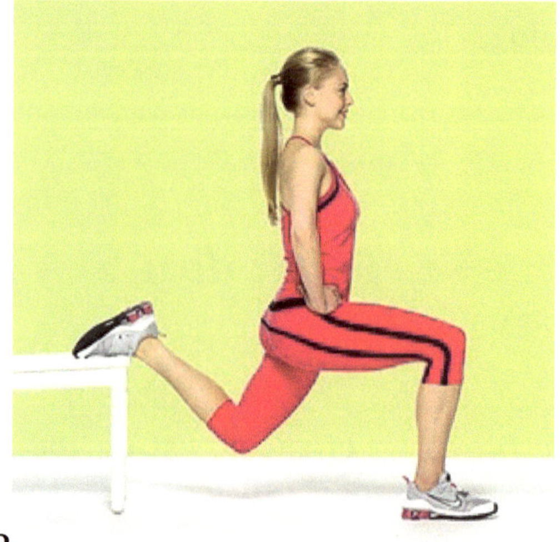

2

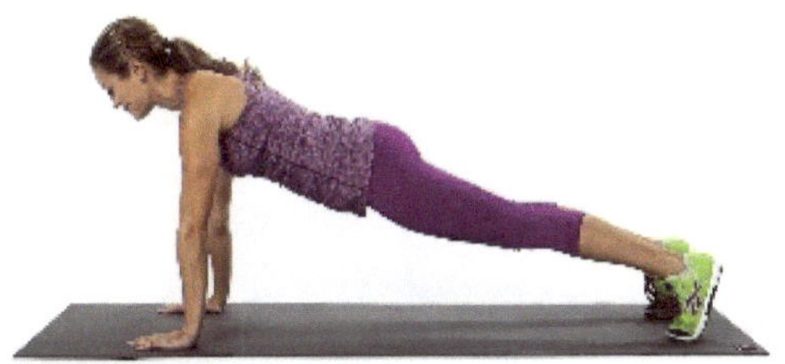

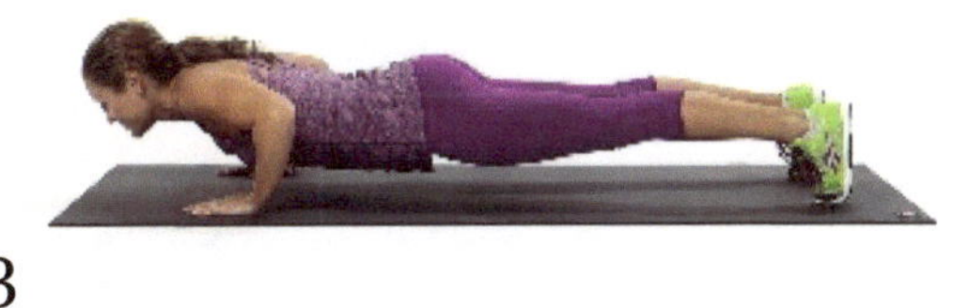

3

Second block: **_3 circles, rest between circles 30 sec_**

5 Reverse crunches 30 rep

6 Plank hip dips 30 rep

7 Hip raises 40 rep

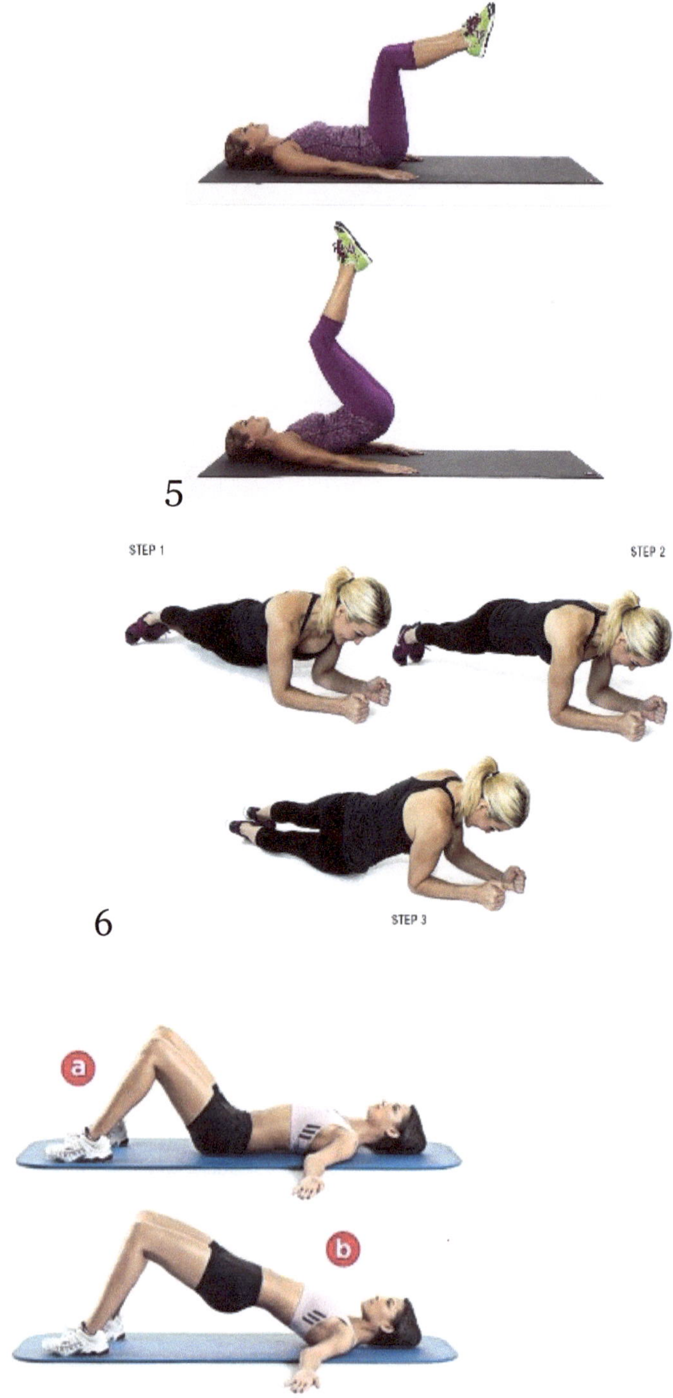

5

6

7

Menu day 10

(menu at 1400-1500 kcal)

For breakfast: 200 grams of milk buckwheat porridge with a baked apple and cinnamon and garnished with a cup of tea with lemon.

For lunch: a glass of yogurt + 1 banana.

For dinner: soup (200g), low-fat mashed potatoes with vegetables (200-250g)

For snack: chicken steak 150 g + tomato + 1 piece of whole-grain bread

For supper: portioned baked fish (150 g), stewed cabbage (150-200 gr)

Exercises for Today
Warm-up

First block: 3 circles, rest between circles 30 sec, between blocks – 1 min

1 Plank into squats 20 rep

2 Squats 25 rep

3 Donkey kicks 40 rep (20 on each leg)

4 Plank 30 sec

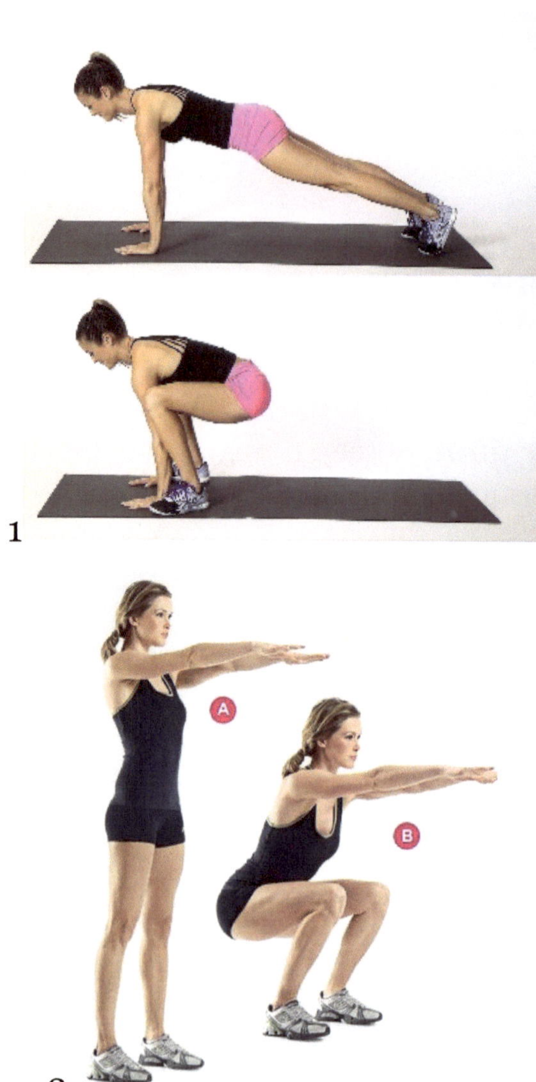

1

2

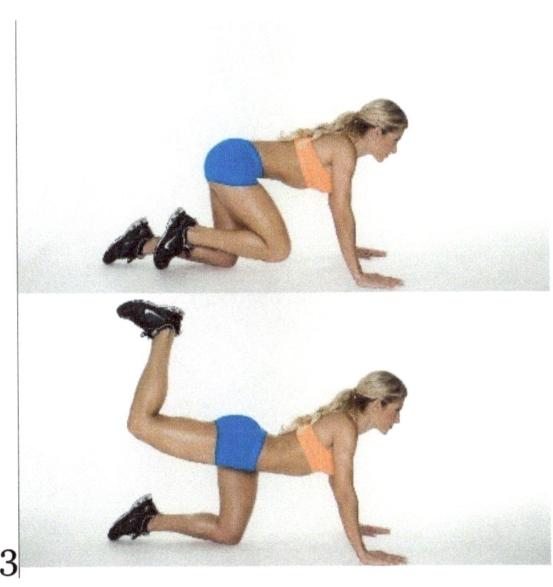

3

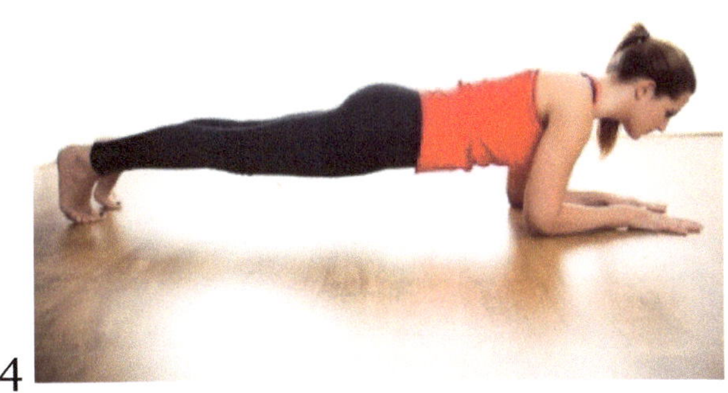

4

Second block: **_3 circles, rest between circles 30 sec_**

5 Crunches 30 rep

6 Bicycle crunches 30 rep

7 Side plank with hip dips 30 rep (15 rep on each leg)

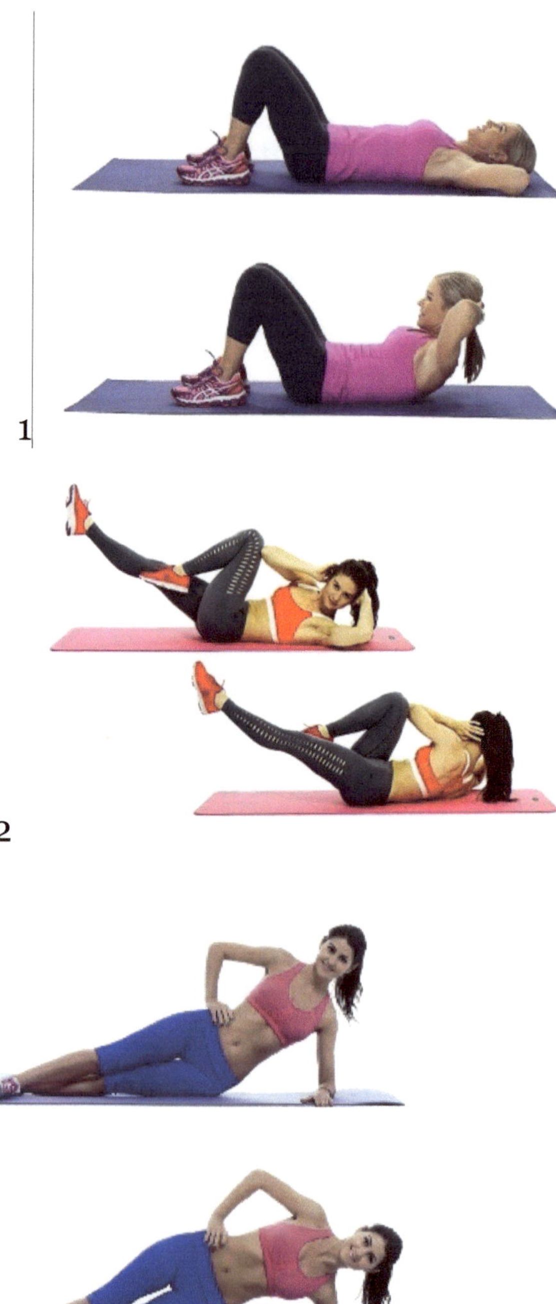

1

2

3

Menu day 11

(menu at 1400-1500 kcal)

For breakfast: fried eggs with 200 g of beans, garnished with a 30g dry oatmeal and about 25g of nuts

For lunch: yogurt with fruit 150 g

For dinner: jelly with 250 g of chicken fillet, eaten with rice with some vegetables weighing about 250 g

For afternoon snack: a toast of black bread with a slice of low-calorie cheese

For supper: turkey with 200g of broccoli

Exercises for Today

Warm-up

First block: 3 circles, rest between circles 30 sec, between blocks – 1 min

1 Running on the spot with the high raising of knees 30 sec

2 Reverse lunge knee-up 40 rep (20 on each leg)

3 Up down plank 20 rep

4 Plie squat jumps 20 rep

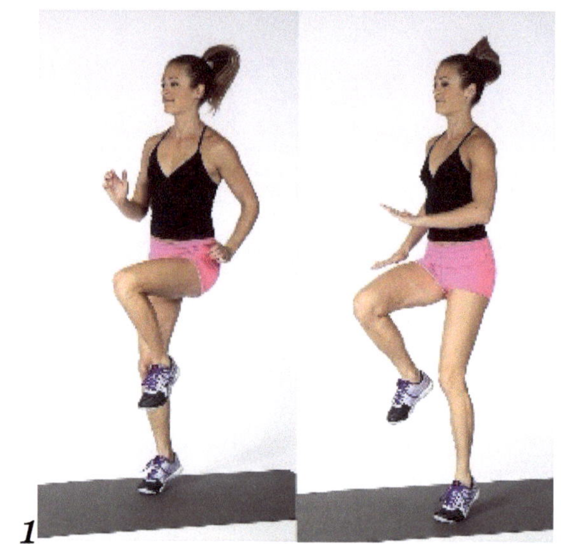

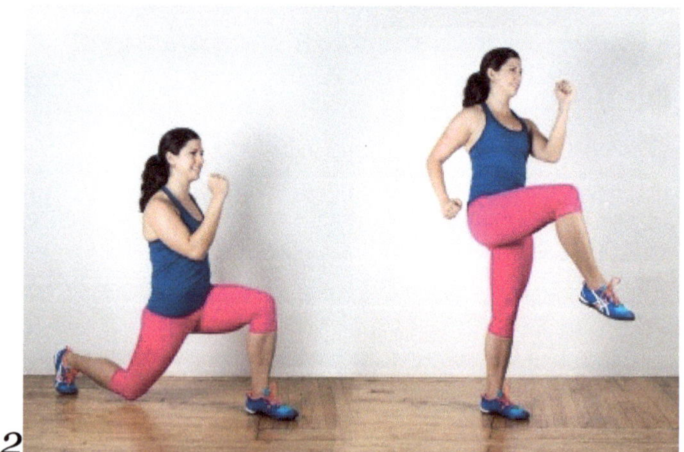

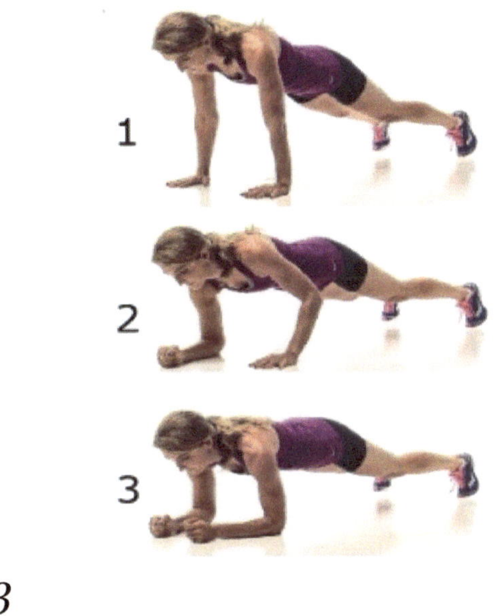

3

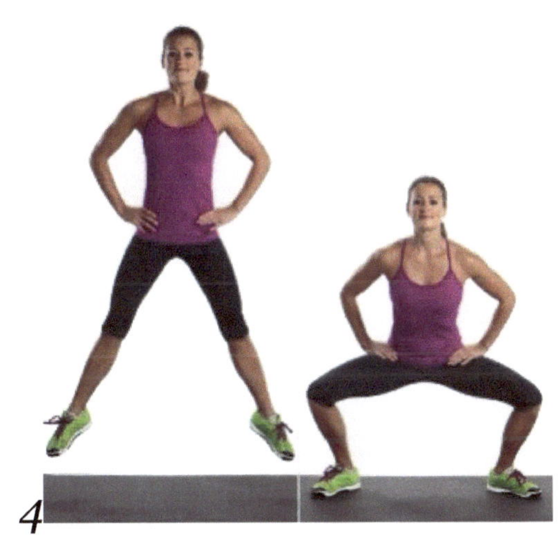

Second block: *3 circles, rest between circles 30 sec*

5 A toe tough crunches 30 rep

6 Mountain climber crunches 30 rep

7 Standing crossover crunches 40 rep (20 on each leg)

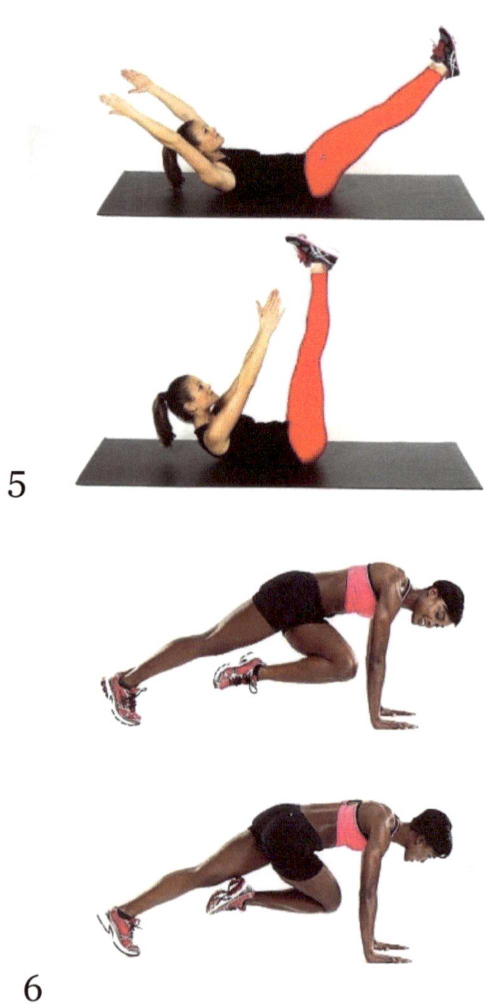

5

6

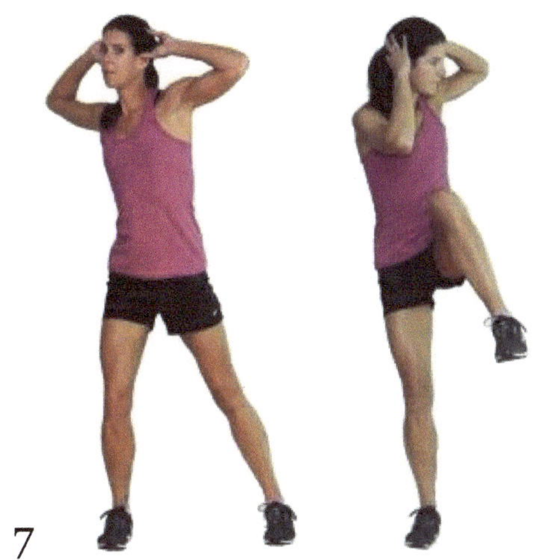

7

The last day of training! Do your best!

Menu day 12

(menu at 1400-1500 kcal)

For breakfast: greek flakes filled with kefir weighing about 150 g, mixed with some 150g of casserole, and taken with a cup of coffee/tea

For lunch: nuts 30 g, apple 1 pc

For dinner: fish soup of about 200 g, mixed with a 100 g of buckwheat and chicken breast weighing about 150 g

For afternoon snack: take about 150g of cottage cheese along with a 30g of raisins

For supper: Salad (broccoli, tomatoes, cucumbers, lettuce, flax seeds) 200 g

Exercises for Today
Warm-up

First block: 3 circles, rest between circles 30 sec, between blocks – 1 min

1 Jump burpees 20 rep

2 Jump lunges 10 rep

3 Plank jacks 25 rep

4 jumping 30 sec

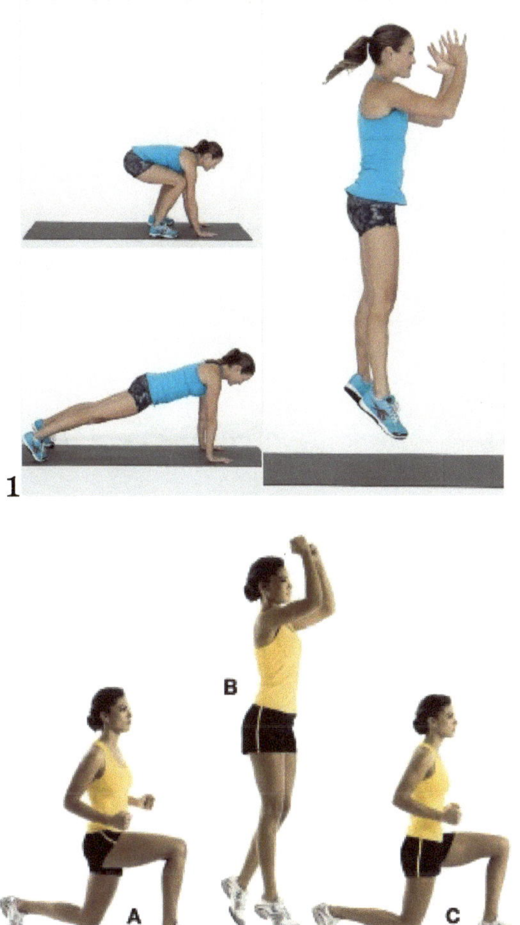

1

2

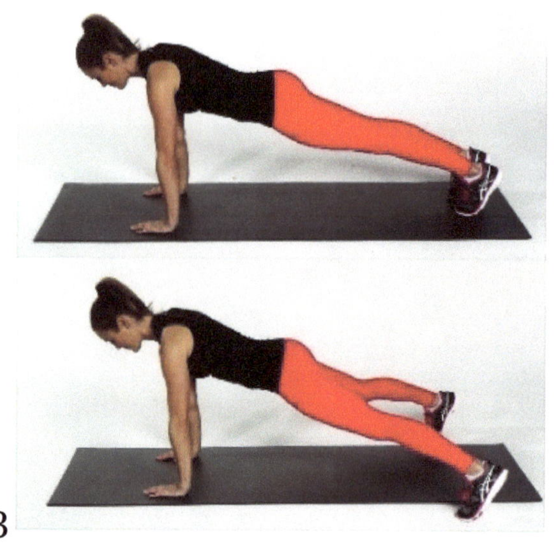

3

Second block: *3 circles, rest between circles 30 sec*

5 Full sit-ups 30 rep

6 Seated knee crunches 30 rep

7 Hyperextension on floor 30 rep

8 Plank 40 sec

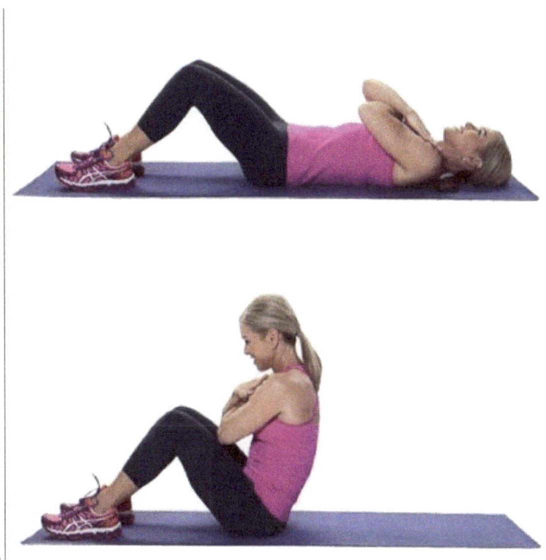

1

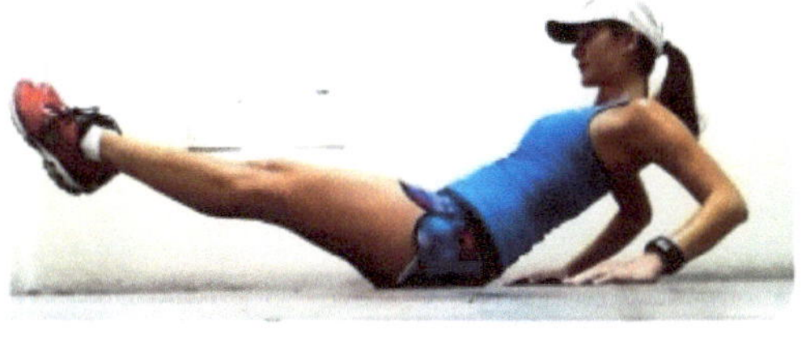

2

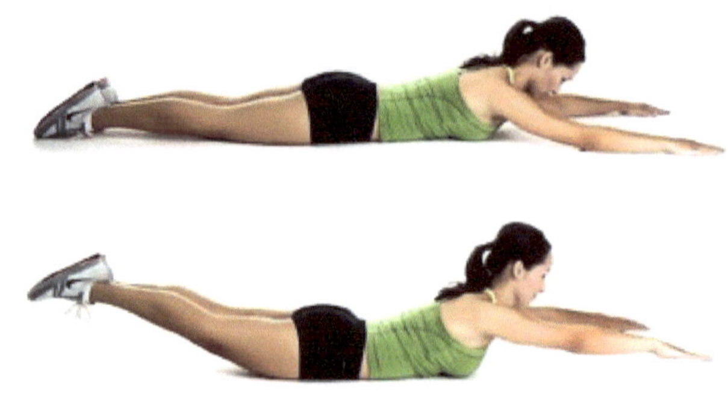

3

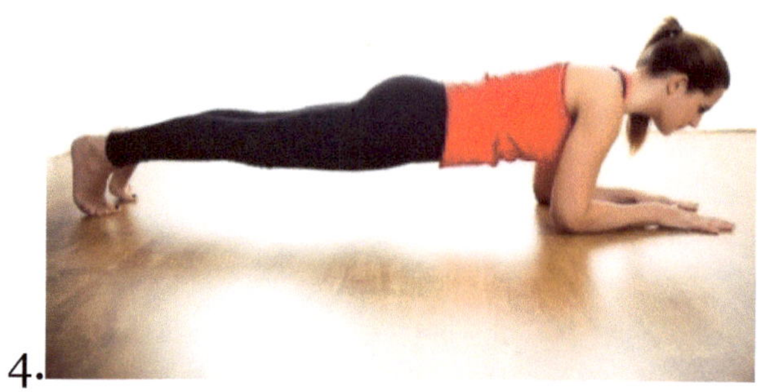

4.

Good job!

I hope the results are visible and they only motivate you to continue.

Sweat now, shine later!

Sandwiches Can Be Useful, And Most Importantly Tasty

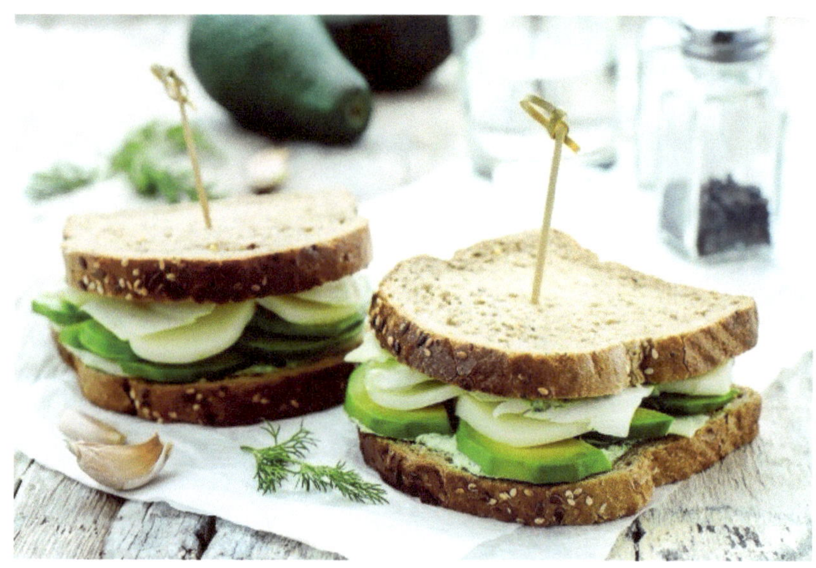

8 options:

- Bread + bacon (grams: 25 + 25, proteins/fats/carbohydrates 6.40 / 8.08 / 11.18, per 100 g: 26.08 / 1.16 / 1.46 / 2.02)

- Bread + cottage cheese + salted salmon, trout, tuna (grams: 25 + 25 + 25, proteins/fats/carbohydrates 12.28 / 4.48 / 11.28, per 100 g: 24.56 / 2.22 / 0.81 / 2.04)

- Bread + beef + mustard + lettuce leaf (grams: 25 + 5 + 25 + 10, proteins/fats/carbohydrates/ 9.04 / 4.89 / 12.31, per 100 g: 23.56 / 1.63 / 0.88 / 2.23)

- Bread + cottage cheese + a plate of pepper + lettuce leaves (grams: 25 + 25 + 25 + 10, proteins/fats/carbohydrates 1,29 / 0,25 / 2,32, per 100 g: 94 / 7,13 / 1, 37 / 12.83)

- Bread + avocado + mozzarella cheese (grams: 25 + 25 + 25, proteins/fats/carbohydrates 7.15 / 9.43 / 12.25, per 100 g: 29.62 / 1.29 / 1.70 / 2.22)

- Bread + cottage cheese + herbs (grams: 25 + 25 + 5, proteins/fats/carbohydrates 6,78 / 1,38 / 11,48, per 100 g: 1,23 / 0,25 / 2,08

- Bread + cottage cheese with sugar substitute + grated carrots (grams: 25 + 25 + 25, proteins/fats/carbohydrates 1.26 / 0.25 / 2.32, per 100 g: 98 / 6.98 / 1.38 / 12.83)

- Bread + boiled minced meat from chicken, mixed with pineapple (grams: 25 + 25 + 25, proteins/fats/carbohydrates 8.55 / 0.90 / 13.85, per 100 g: 17.78 / 1.55 / 0.16 / 2.50)

15 Options For Proper Protein Suppers

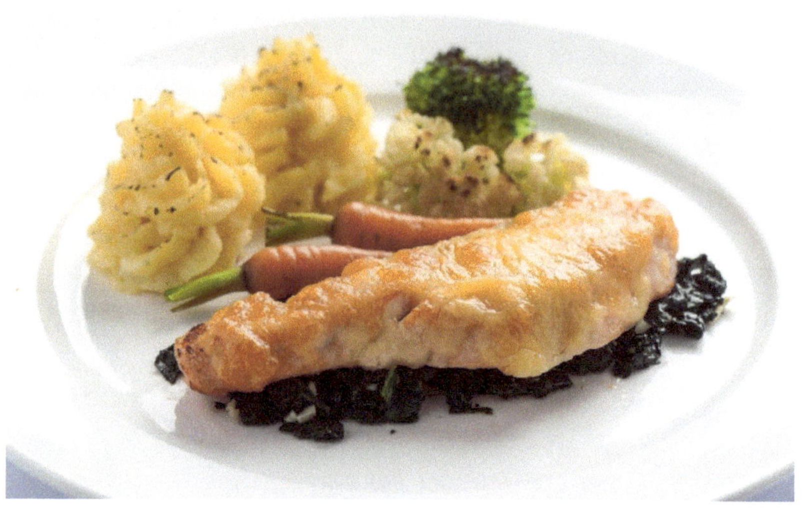

1. Eat a typical omelet, created from a mixture of egg and milk. Garnish it with some fresh tomatoes or vegetables.

2. Roasted chicken fillet flavored in lemon juice with spices and garnished with vegetables.

3. Garnish some vegetables with salmon or any other type of fish.

4. Garnish some meat baked in foil in an oven with some tomato salad sprinkled all over it.

5. Garnish some chicken fillet baked with some spices in a foil.

6. Eat some chicken soup or some seafood. However, desist from combining it with some soup meant for dinners such as potatoes, meat, and cereals.

7. Salad of vegetables and tuna in its own juice.

8. Fish or chicken cutlets baked in the oven.

9. 200 g cottage cheese with cinnamon.

10. Garnish some boiled Pollock and cooked beans together.

11. Eat some vegetable sauce mixed with some braised veal.

12. Salad with chicken breast and celery.

13. Salad from a mixture of lettuce leaves and mozzarella cheese.

14. Turkey fillet, baked in foil, and a garnish of fresh greens and cucumber.

15. Seabass baked on a vegetable cushion.

10 Rations From A Nutritionist At 1400-1600 Kcal

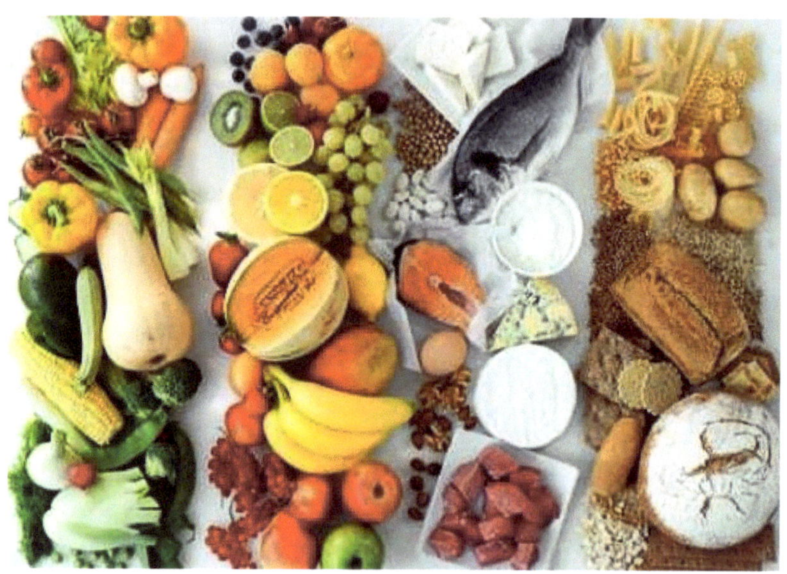

1.

For breakfast: buckwheat porridge with milk 200 g, egg 1 pc, coffee/tea

For snack: banana 1pc

For dinner: rice 200 g, chicken fillet with vegetables 200 g

For afternoon snack: Greek yogurt 100 g, nuts 25 g

For supper: cauliflower baked with cheese (low-fat) 200g

2.

For breakfast: egg 1 pc, oatmeal 30 g (dry), whole-grain bread 1 pc, cheese 25 g

For snack: nuts 30 g, yogurt 100 g

For dinner: buckwheat 150 g, chicken fillet with vegetables 200 g

For afternoon snack: apple 1 pc, whole-grain bread 1 pc, cheese 25 g

For supper: cottage cheese 150 g

3.

For breakfast: 200 g, 1 egg, coffee/tea

For snack: fruit salad 150 g

For dinner: rice 200 g, fish 150 g, vegetable salad 150 g

For afternoon snack: Greek yogurt 150 g, whole-grain bread 1 pc

For supper: vegetable stew 200 g, braised chicken 150 g

4.

For breakfast: oatmeal with raisins and nuts 100 g, omelet with two eggs, coffee/tea

For snack: cottage cheese with fruit 200 g

For dinner: broccoli, baked with low-fat cheese 200 g, chicken fillet with vegetables 150 g

For afternoon snack: kefir 200 g

For supper: fish pollack with vegetables 200 g

5.

For breakfast: eggs from two eggs, milk rice porridge 200 g, coffee/tea

For snack: yogurt greek 200 g, fruit 100 g

For dinner: rice noodles with vegetables 250 g, mushroom soup 250 g

For afternoon snack: pistachios 30 g

For supper: baked salmon 250 g

6.

For breakfast: oatmeal porridge 50 g (dry), cottage cheese pancakes 150 g, a spoon of honey, coffee/tea

For snack: nuts 30 g, apple 1 pc

For dinner: rice 150 g, pink salmon, cooked in oven 200 g, vegetable salad 150 g

For afternoon snack: egg 1 piece, vegetables 150 g

For supper: boiled chicken breast 200 g, baked vegetables 150 g

7.

For breakfast: pancakes zucchini 150 g, egg 1 piece, whole grain bread 50 g

For snack: baked apple with cottage cheese 1 pc, yogurt with fruit 150 g

For dinner: vegetable soup 200 g, salmon baked in foil 150 g, vegetable salad 100 g

For afternoon snack: banana 1 piece, cottage cheese 100 g

For supper: chicken boiled 150 g, vegetable salad 100 g